Home Remedies and Natural Cures

Effective Home Remedies For Many Of Your Common Ailments

Written by
Jade Flannery

"Let your food be your medicine and your medicine your food."

--Hippocrates

Table of Contents

Introduction

For those of you, who hate running to the doctor for every cough and sneeze, find themselves wondering everywhere for the best home remedies for their condition. Many people choose to go the home remedy route of treatment due to the fact that home remedies are less likely to cause side effects like prescription medications do.

Many people don't know that a lot of the prescriptions that we receive for illnesses or conditions cause more harm to our bodies than good. Another thing that many people don't know is that taking antibiotics for long periods of time can ultimately make your body susceptible to any antibiotics.

For a lot of people, some antibiotics don't clear up all of the symptoms they are suffering from and they find themselves run back to the doctor for another dose and then another and another, etc. This is mainly because their body is now used to the antibiotics being ingested and simply don't do anything in the treatment of your symptoms you are enduring.

Taking certain antibiotics can also cause a super infection to form. Many studies have shown that prescription medications simply don't work for many illnesses and conditions and have major side effects associated with them.

Home remedies are not only natural and beneficial but also helps treat a lot of illnesses and conditions quicker than any antibiotic. Many of the home remedies that you will find in this book have been used for many years and have been tested and proven to work.

Keep in mind that home remedies will not cure all illnesses and conditions and if your symptoms persist for more than 5-7 days then you will need to consult with your physician for further testing and treatment. You also need to keep in mind that a lot of people have many different allergies to certain things, so make sure before you try a home remedy that you are not allergic to any of the ingredients or home remedies that you test.

I have researched the top illnesses and conditions that most people are looking for and have compiled them all into one book, all with the most popular and most commonly used home remedies to treat their symptoms.

So what are you waiting for? Start reading now… and start treating yourself the health and natural way through the top used home remedies today!

Acid Reflux

Who wants to deal with the pain and discomfort of acid reflux? Not me… and probably not you either. Although there are a lot of over the counter medications that you can take for acid reflux, they can be a very expensive and sometimes not even a useful treatment option. Why pay tons of money when there are simple home remedies that can allow you to eat those spicy foods you always have to avoid. Try these helpful home remedies and watch your worries of acid reflux diminish.

Baking Soda, Water, & Lemon Juice – this has got to be about the best and most used home remedy for your acid reflux. In this home remedy you simply put 2 tablespoons of baking soda into a tall glass, fill your glass about half full with cold water, you then pour the juice of one freshly squeezed lemon into your glass, and drink the mixture as quick as possible. I would advise that when mixing all of the ingredients that you do this over a kitchen sink as the baking soda and water will fizz and will tower over your glass. However, that is why this mixture should be consumed very quickly, because it is the fizz and water that will provide you the relief from your acid reflux.

BE ADVISED that is you have a history or have been diagnosed with hypertension (high blood pressure) you do not want to try this home remedy. This is because the remedy itself will create sodium in your system.

Apple Cider Vinegar – is another highly popular home remedy for the relief of your acid reflux. Apple cider vinegar is believed to work so well due to the fact that the acidity of the vinegar mocks as the acid in your stomach helping to make it easier to digest the food that you have consumed. Simply take one tablespoon of apple cider vinegar and mix it with about 3/4 of a cup of water. If you have a hard time stomaching this mixture, you can also add a teaspoon of sugar or honey to the mixture to make it a bit more tolerable for you.

Regardless of the taste of the mixture this home remedy is one of the leading remedies for instant acid reflux relief. Just simply take this mixture before a meal or during a meal for best results. If you suffer from acid reflux at night, you can also consume the mixture right before bed and rest assure that you won't be woke up during the night with the hassles of acid reflux again! You can purchase apple cider vinegar in a pill form also, although the juice mixture is more effective and is absorbed by your body better.

Aloe Vera – oh yea, that's right aloe vera and I don't mean the lotion! Many people aren't aware that aloe vera is also found in a juice form. The juice provides you with the very same cooling effect that the lotion treatment gives you and it will help reduce the amount of acid in your stomach. You can simply drink anywhere from 1-2 ounces of the aloe vera juice and provide yourself with instant relief as well as a drop in the frequency of your acid reflux. If you do choose to take this treatment option, you will not want to take it more than once a day.

Raw Potato Juice – who would have thought that a raw potato keep be the answers to all of your acid reflux problems... but it can... believe it or not! Raw potato juice is proven to prevent over buildup of acid in your stomach from the consumption of acidic foods. The raw potato juice method has been used for many years and used to be used by boiling a raw potato (unpeeled) for several hours before drinking. However, studies have shown that actually juicing the potato yourself is not only a quicker method but is also more potent. You simply wash the potato (do not peel the potato), juice the raw potato with a standard juicer, and then mix the raw potato juice with equal amounts of water. You will want to consume this mixture immediately and you will find yourself free of your acid reflux discomfort. You can follow this method up to 3-4 times a day and should be used as needed.

Pineapple Juice or Fresh Pineapple – yes, not only can raw vegetables be your friend, but some fruits also. Pineapples have proved to be great acid reducers. Pineapples are packed with tons of enzymes and contain bromelain. These particular enzymes are the exact enzymes that also help with the reduction of acid in your stomach. Bromelain provide you with digestion support and also reduces inflammation (swelling), which is a big factor in stopping your acid reflux symptoms. Because pineapples and pineapple juice are natural fruits, there is no limit on how many you consume. Keep in mind that the juice form of the pineapple is the best and quickest treatment for your acid reflux.

Chewing Gum – so I know you have heard the phrase of a person who, "can't chew bubblegum and walk at the same time," right? Well I don't know about walking… but you can certainly chew bubble gum and start reducing your acid reflux! Yes, I know it sounds crazy, but there is a science to the madness of this theory. Chewing gum produces mega amounts of saliva and your saliva is a natural antacid. So when you are chewing the gum, your saliva will neutralize any of the acid that is in your stomach and any acid that is coming up your esophagus. Try this and you might find your road to an acid reflux free life.

Herbal Teas – There are certain types of herbal teas that will also help you in your journey to an acid reflux free life. Teas that consist of peppermint, lavender, and anise have also been known to cure many acid reflux cases. Rather than buying premade herbal teas (which may not contain these specific herbs), try purchasing the specific herbs and making the tea mixture yourself. To make the tea you will first need to put equal amounts of each herb into one cup. You can use anywhere from 1-2 tablespoons of each herb. Then you will add boiling distilled water to the mixture. Mix this altogether and you have created yourself immediate acid reflux relief. Drinking at least 8 ounces up to two times a day you will find that there is a major decrease in your acid reflux episodes.

Ginger or Ginger Root – can also help you with your acid reflux discomfort. Ginger has the ability to absorb acid... which is very good news for you if you suffer with acid reflux. Ginger is very easily found in the spice isle of your grocery store. Ginger and ginger root has been used for many, many years and studies have shown that ginger is great for digestion, which is why it makes it so powerful when it comes to acid in your stomach. You can also purchase ginger raw (in root form), and can also be consumed raw. You will soon find that incorporating ginger or ginger root into your diet, can be a major perk for the reduction of acid. Note that ginger should however be taken in small amounts when you are trying this method for acid reflux relief.

Useful Treatment Tips

➢ Drinking pickle juice can also provide you with acid reflux relief. Pickle juice contains vinegar which is a leading ingredient used to mimic your stomach acids. So if you can stomach drinking straight pickle juice, you will find that this is an excellent acid reducer.

➢ Eating a slender piece of celery before and after meals can also give you instant acid reflux relief. Some find this method to be very beneficial and also very healthy.

➢ There are certain foods that are good for your acid reflux... as well as there are foods that are bad for your acid reflux. You always want to start by eating a healthy diet consisting of vegetables and fruits. You will want to make sure that the meats that you eat are not cooked in too much fat and you will want to avoid chocolate and alcoholic beverages. Eating foods such as almonds, bananas, peppermint, figs, and papaya before you go to bed at night can greatly prevent the occurrence of your acid reflux.

➢ You can also make a tea with chamomile or lavender. Simmer one teaspoon of licorice root powder for about 15 minutes in a pan with one cup of water. Add one teaspoon of chamomile or lavender and then cover it and let it stand for about 15 minutes. You will however need to use a strainer to strain the mixture. You will want to drink the mixture while it is still warm.

Anxiety

Anxiety is a common condition that a lot of people suffer with each day. The most common sign of anxiety is having an anxiety attack. Some of the most common symptoms related to anxiety are tightening of the chest, shortness of breath, unwanted thoughts and worries, and periods of hot flashes. Anxiety attacks can potentially take over a person's life with. However, there are some home remedies that can help your anxiety symptoms that are natural and have been tested and proven to help a person with their anxiety dramatically.

Good Sleeping Habits – Make sure that you are getting enough sleep. Not having enough sleep can lead a person to having many of the anxiety symptoms and will only intensify them. Getting 3 hours here and 4 hours there is not healthy for anyone, especially for someone suffering with bouts of anxiety. Make sure that you are getting the required 6-9 hours of sleep to better help with your health as well as starting you off to a better outlook on the day as a whole and a better more refreshed attitude.

Getting a Breath of Fresh Air – In this particular home remedy you will need to practice deep breathing. Most commonly people breathe quickly and shallow which then creates stress hormones. The shallow breathing is one of the symptoms that are most associated with anxiety attacks. However, with some time outside and a nice breath of fresh air you can help and even eventually alleviate anxiety attacks all together. Try taking 20 minutes out of your daily routine devoted to meditation, preferably during the morning and then once again in the evening. This will give you what studies have shown to be called a relaxation response. It does take a couple sessions of meditation before your body starts to respond. However, the more times that you meditate on a regular basis the more your body and mind will become familiar with the practice and be more noticeable to the effects of meditation. The key thing to remember is that you want to make yourself as relaxed as possible and in the right breathing pattern. Using breathe as a focus point in your meditation also helps with adding oxygen into your body which can not only help you feel at peace but also will enhance your meditation experience.

Therapeutic Baths – This home remedy has been used for many years and originated first in Japan. Therapeutic baths have been tested and proven to be one of the best ways to gain relaxation. Run some soothing lukewarm bathwater and then add some aroma therapy, and a natural bubble bath with incense. You can also use candles with aroma scents and place them around your bath tub while you are relaxing. You can also add a few drops of lavender essential oils and also gain some relaxation and also helps you get a goodnight rest.

Exercise – can be a great way to relieve some stress. Aerobic exercise is one of the top forms of exercise that relieves and reduces your stress level. Not only will you feel better about yourself and give you positive thoughts, but it also helps you in your breathing patterns.

Incorporating good exercise in your daily routine can help you dramatically with your anxiety symptoms.

Oranges – It has been tested and proven that just the scent alone of an orange can lower your anxiety level. Simply take the peels from an orange and place them in a pan of water and boil for just a few minutes and then let the mixture simmer on your stove. This creates a very comforting aroma for you and your home as well because the orange peels will release calming, fragranced oil. Try using this method periodically and watch your anxiety diminish away to nothing.

Almonds – Almonds have also been proven to help with anxiety related symptoms. Taking around 10 almonds and soaking them overnight in water, then peeling the skins and putting the almonds in a blender with one cup of warm milk, creates a tasty treat and a stress reliever cocktail. You can also add about a half of a teaspoon of nutmeg and a half of a teaspoon of ginger to this concoction to create another relaxing infusion. The best time to drink the cocktail is at night before going to bed. You will wake up feeling refreshed and less stressed as well as ready for the next day's daily activities.

Chamomile – Grabbing some herbal tea with chamomile in it can also help with your nerves and with your sleeping at night. You can also create a chamomile tea yourself by taking a tablespoon of chamomile flowers and steep them in about a cup of hot water for about 15-20 minutes. Make sure to breathe the aroma as the mixture is cooling which will give you a relaxing feeling. Then strain the mixture and drink your herbal chamomile tea.

Useful Treatment Tips

> ➢ You can also try getting a massage and add a little sesame oil to the mix to help with relaxation also. Simply heat up around 6 ounces of sesame oil until the mixture is warm. You can also use coconut or corn oil and receive the same results as using sesame oil. Once the oil has warmed you then rub the oil all over your body... even your scalp. This will give you an incredible sense of relaxation and calming. This can also be used if you are having trouble with loss of sleep due to anxiety by applying the oil to your body before you go to bed.

> ➢ Baking soda can also help calm your nerves and relax your body. Simply add 1/3 of a cup of baking soda and about 1/3 of a cup of ginger to your warm bath water. Take a relaxing bath in this mixture for around 15-20 minutes and you will see noticeable change in your relaxation state instantly. This is a very good method to relieve stress, anxiety, and tension.

> ➢ You can also try an herb called passion flower if you are having problems with sleeping due to your anxiety symptoms. This is normally found in health and nutritional stores and should not be taken with a sedative unless under medical supervision. This herb acts as a medication for sleep as well as seizure

disorders. Make sure to check the labels to make sure that this is right for you.

Cholesterol

Having high cholesterol can be a scary situation. Cholesterol is the wax like substance present in cell walls, arteries, and other membranes in your body. A high build-up of cholesterol on your arteries can cause blockages which restrains blood flow to the artery, causing the possibility of a heart attack or stroke. Knowing this, it is very important that you try to lower your cholesterol to prevent these conditions from happening. Keep in mind that there are three different cholesterol levels, LDL or bad cholesterol, HDL or good cholesterol, and triglycerides and you need to get these levels checked periodically, especially if you have high cholesterol or a history of low cholesterol. Other than using a treatment plan consisting of medication, there are also some dietary home remedies that you can try as well to help lower your cholesterol.

Almonds, Honey, and Beets – Almonds have shown to dramatically reduce your LDL cholesterol. By making almonds apart of your diet can decrease your cholesterol as much as 10 percent. Try snacking on some almonds periodically during the day and watch your levels start changing for the good. Honey has also been proven to decrease your LDL cholesterol. Simply add one teaspoon of honey and one teaspoon of lime juice to a hot glass of water each morning and you'll see what a difference it makes on your cholesterol in the long run. Beets are a great addition to your diet when trying to decrease your cholesterol levels. Beets are filled with flavonoids and carotenoids which are two components that help decrease the build-up of cholesterol on your arteries. You can eat beets fresh or canned. However, studies have shown that eating fresh beets decrease your cholesterol at a faster rate as well as more effective.

Olive Oil, Oats, and Walnuts – Olive oil has also been proven to help you you're your cholesterol. Studies have shown that olive oil is also a good source of dramatically increasing your levels of HDL and also lower levels of LDL which will prevent your blood from forming clots in your arteries. Oats are also very effective in fighting off cholesterol problems. Why not try eating a bowl of oatmeal every morning for breakfast to lower your cholesterol. Make sure to eat oats in raw form, studies have also shown that eating oats in raw form has proven to be more effective in diminishing cholesterol from forming. Along with almonds, walnuts are also a very good source and snack to help prevent the build-up of cholesterol. Eating walnuts at least 4-6 times a week can lower your cholesterol levels as much as 16 percent.

Garlic and Chicory – Here are two herbal treatments for lowering your cholesterol levels. Garlic has shown to reduce the amount of fat that is in your blood, along with lowering your LDL cholesterol and raising your HDL cholesterol. Using garlic in raw form as well as powdered form can both be useful, although consuming garlic in raw form has been proven to be more effective. Using anywhere from one tablespoon to two tablespoons per day in your meals at least 4-5 times a week can dramatically decrease your LDL cholesterol by as much as 12 percent.

Chicory has also shown to lower your levels of cholesterol. Chicory is an herb that is normally added to your tea while brewing. Consuming between 1-2 cups of chicory tea a day will definitely do the trick and you will see your cholesterol levels start dropping each and every time your cholesterol levels are checked. Chicory can be found most commonly in the spice isle in your local grocery store. You can also purchase herbal tea brews that contain chicory and can also lower your cholesterol level, however using the actual spice has proven to work more effectively.

Below are a few more home remedies that you can use for the treatment of high cholesterol.

Useful Treatment Tips

> ➢ Boiling 10 cinnamon sticks in about 6 cups of water and then adding one tablespoon of honey can mix up to be a powerful mixture to fight bad cholesterol from forming. Make sure that when you consume the mixture that you consume the mixture hot.

> ➢ Soy products, artichokes, and yogurt has also been proven to lower levels of LDL cholesterol. By consuming any one of these items at least 2-3 times a week can help lower your levels intensely. Soy products are also very rich in isoflavones which can effectively regulate your cholesterol levels.

> ➢ Drinking 8-10 glasses of water can also bring down your cholesterol. In this home remedy you are

flushing your whole body and the more you have proper excretion from your body, the more you will see your cholesterol levels diminish.

➤ You can also try boiling 2 tablespoons of coriander seeds in a glass of water and create an infusion to lower your cholesterol as well as regulate your levels. You will however find better results by consuming at least 2-3 glasses of the mixture a day to see your cholesterol levels start to drop.

➤ Consuming vitamin B6 and vitamin E can also help to regulate your cholesterol levels and lower cholesterol levels also. Vitamin B6 can be found in such food items as yeast and wheat. Vitamin E can be found in such food items as sunflower seeds, grains, soy bean oil, and sprouted seeds.

➤ The intake of onion juice can also become an effective treatment for high cholesterol. The onion not only lowers your cholesterol, but also helps clean your blood and regulates your heart.

➤ Consuming food items such as wholegrain cereals, egg yolks, soybeans, and vegetable oil that contain lechithin are a big cholesterol fighter.

Common Cold

More and more people are finding themselves using home remedies rather than going to the doctor and taking medication after medication for the common cold. There are many home remedies that you can try to cure symptoms related to the common cold and many of the remedies have been used for more than 100 years. The best part is that all of the ingredients can most commonly be found in your homes already.

Many of the top home remedy ingredients can be found in your pantries, refrigerators, or in a linen closet. Not only are these ingredients readily available to you... but you also save yourself a co-pay on a doctor's visit as well as a co-pay on the medication prescribed for your cold. Most people don't know that the more you take a medication the more susceptible your body becomes to the medications the less effective the drug will be. This is why many people have turned to old fashioned home remedies to cure their common cold symptoms. Here are a few home remedies that you use to cure a common cold:

Chicken Noodle Soup - I'm pretty sure everyone has been advised at least one time in their life when they have had a cold to eat chicken noodle soup. Chicken noodle soup is a great home remedy to use for a common cold and can ease your symptoms associated with a common cold. Chicken noodle soup contains an ingredient called selenium, this ingredient is important because it helps with the function of your immune system as well as for overall good health.

Chicken noodle soup is most commonly served warm. The warm soup helps soothe the throat and the steam from the soup can also help with nasal decongestion and opening up your breathing airways. This makes it easier for a person with a cold to breathe. You can also add different spices to your chicken noodle soup that also helps in cold symptoms, such as garlic, pepper, and onions. These common spices can help the effectiveness of the treatment of your symptoms for your common cold. These spices are also good additions to your chicken noodle soup because you can taste and smell these spices, which are most commonly diminished during the course of the cold. Chicken noodle soup has been recommended for ages and is proved to be a very common home remedy for the common cold.

Honey, Lemon Juice, & Other Herbal Teas - Many common colds can also be cured by many different herbal teas as well as lemon juice and honey. There are various reasons why each help with the symptoms of a common cold. Lemon juice contains vitamin C, which is very important for the function of your immune system. Using herbal teas that contain mullein work very good when sweetened with honey and lemon juice. All of these ingredients incorporated together can sooth your throat as well as temporarily unclog your breathing airways.

You can also pour and mix honey and lemon juice together and take tablespoons periodically during the course of your cold and this will ease your cold symptoms such as your throat and breathing. Preparing your favorite tea and replacing the sugar with honey can also help with these symptoms. You can also boil two cups of water with a half of a lemon. Once the tea is prepared you can sweeten this tea by using either honey or sugar. Small children however, should not use or be given honey. To help relieve coughing you can also use a tea called horehound tea. You can also increase your energy as well as metabolism with green tea.

Orange Juice, Gatorade, Sprite, & Pedialyte - Using the helpful source of orange juice can also help with your troubling cold symptoms. Orange juice provides you with a great source of vitamin C, which is a leading vitamin to getting you back on your feet again. Whenever you are feeling sick, doctors always recommend keeping fluids in your body. What better fluid then one that allow you to absorb vitamin C as well. Vitamin C, as studies have shown, is also used to improve your immune system functions, which is the number one thing you want to keep in tip top shape if you are more prone to catching colds. However, do not use orange juice if you have an upset stomach. The acid from the orange juice will only make it worse on you and your stomach.

In a case where your stomach is upset and you are not able to consume anything acidic, using Gatorade, Sprite, and Pedialyte can be handy and useful. Gatorade, as well as Pedialyte, helps in the restoration of electrolytes in your body. Often, diarrhea and vomiting occurs with upset stomachs, and the consumption of foods is just not an option. In this case, Gatorade and Pedialyte can still give your body the nutrients it needs to fight viruses as well as keep your body hydrated. Keeping fluids in your body is one of the top things to keep in mind if you are not able to consume anything solid. Dehydration will only make matters worse for both you and your body.

Humidifiers and Steam Baths – Humidifiers are commonly used with common colds that involve congestion, as well as steam baths. Inhaling steam can not only open your airways but also help you in a speedy recovery from your cold. Placing a humidifier in a small concealed room can trap the steam and help dry out your nasal cavities. You can also add aromatherapy in the mix of things. Using scents such as cinnamon, peppermint, and Vicks Vapor Solution can not only open your airways but also provide you with an easier more comfortable rest. You can also add these scents to hot bath water giving the shower steam the same effect as a humidifier. You can also add lavender oil to your bath and this will help with decongestion as well as help you with a smoother more relaxed sleep. Using tea tree oil as well as lemon oils, and this will also provide you with the same relief. You can also try taking a foot bath with mustard in it. I know it sounds crazy, but it really does help in nasal decongestion, as well as those clogged up breathing passages. Some experts believe that using a humidifier or a steam shower is not good for getting rid of the infection and doesn't relieve common cold symptoms. They believe that a dry nose only leads to making you more susceptible to viral infections. Researchers have found that the rhinovirus and other viruses are more active in lower humidity, which is why people are more common to getting a cold in the winter months rather than the warmer months. However, viruses thrive on more moist and hot conditions that are most commonly always present in your nose. In my opinion and my own experiences, I do however believe that humidifiers as well as steam baths help greatly in clearing up congestion and making your sleeping habits more tolerable.

Useful Treatment Tips

> Eating ginger can help encourage sweating and can also help sooth your aching throat. Simply take 2 teaspoons of ginger powder and boil it in a cup of water, then add about a ½ teaspoon of sugar. This mixture should be consumed very warm in temperature. You can also add ginger to your herbal teas and it can act as a fever reducer. You can do these procedures up to two times a day.

> Ginseng can also be added to your tea to help support your immune system as well as helps your body to fight off infections at a faster rate.

> Garlic can act as an antiseptic as well as carries antispasmodic properties. The oil from the garlic opens up your airway passages. Garlic has also been proven to reduce a fever dramatically! You can try this by making a garlic soup which consists of 3-4 cloves of chopped garlic placed into a cup of boiling water. Garlic soup flushes out all of the toxins that are in your airway passages, which helps drop your temperature if you have a fever.

➢ Turmeric can also help with the irritation of your throat. Simply take a half of a teaspoon of turmeric powder and mix it in 1/8 cup of warm milk at least one to two times a day to ease the irritation of your throat.

➢ If you have a dry or stuffy nose you can try using saline or salt water nasal drops. You can do this by adding 1/4 of a teaspoon of table salt and a teaspoon of lukewarm water. Using a clean dropper you can drop 1-2 drops in each nostril anywhere from 3-4 times a day. Keep this mixture in the fridge and you will want to make a new mixture every couple of days until your symptoms subside.

Constipation

Constipation is a very common condition that even the healthiest of people can acquire. This can also be a very uncomfortable condition and sometimes painful. Other than using laxatives that have many side effects, many people opt in to using a more natural way to cure their constipation. They can do this through using natural home remedies. Here is some of the most popular home remedies used for the treatment of constipation.

Water – Although this home remedy may sound too simple to be true, it is. Drinking an adequate amount of water can both help prevent constipation as well as treat your constipation. You will need to drink at least 8 glasses of water each day to insure that things are running smoothly throughout your body. However, when you find yourself with occasional constipation increasing your levels of intake on water can dramatically alleviate your constipation and give you the relief you are looking for.

Coffee – Even if you are not a regular coffee drinker, if you are having the pain and discomfort due to constipation, you may find yourself hugging onto a cup of coffee. Coffee, like other items of food that consist of the bitter taste, naturally stimulates your digestive system which can ultimately alleviate your constipation. Make sure to drink your coffee lukewarm as this will relax your digestive system also and helps the natural flow of your digestive track.

Honey – is a fast acting ingredient that can help kick your digestive system into overdrive. Honey is a very mild ingredient and can be taken straight from a tablespoon or it can also be mixed in your favorite drink or herbal tea. You can also mix 2 tablespoons of honey with about a cup of warm water and also get the same relief.

Molasses – is very similar to honey, however, it can be bit harsher for your taste buds. Nonetheless, molasses has been used for ages in the cure of constipation in individuals all across the world. Simply take 2 tablespoons of blackstrap molasses and mix it into milk or to fruit juice. Mixing the molasses with milk or fruit juice will mild the general taste of molasses and make it more tolerable to ingest. The best way to take this mixture for the best results is to take this before bed so that the ingredients can work throughout the night and by morning time instant relief of constipation for you and your digestive system.

Oil – is also a very handy home remedy when it comes to constipation symptoms. Oils have a lubricating effect that can work to your benefit big time when trying to unclog your digestive track. Look at it like this, when you're cooking you generally use oil to make sure that foods don't stick to pans. This works the same as when you apply this to your digestive system. So this means that the oils unclog virtually anything that was stuck with its natural lubricants. Keep in mind, when using this home remedy the oil does not have to be consumed just straight oil, you can also make it into a salad dressing. Just make sure that you are using a tablespoon at least 2-3 times a day until your constipation has subsided. A great salad dressing mixture to use is by taking 1-2 tablespoons of oil, half of a teaspoon of lemon juice, and herbs of your choice sprinkled in the dressing. Salad dressing is a great option because not only does the oil from the salad dressing work for your digestive system but also the leafy greens in your salad are good for digestion purposes because they hold high properties of fiber. So now your constipation gets a double dose of treatment all in one meal. You will soon find yourself comfortable and pain free from constipation.

Vegetables and Fruits – Fiber is a big factor in relieving constipation symptoms, so what better way to incorporate fiber than eating high in fiber vegetables and fruits. Fiber is excellent in making your digestive system regular and on track with a steady flow. Eating a wide variety of fruits and vegetables should be applied to your meal plan daily and especially in numbers when constipation in present. For best results each the fruit or vegetable as a whole rather than in juice form. Although fruit and vegetable juices contain vitamins, the real whole fruits themselves carry more properties of fiber than fruit and vegetable juices. Fruits and vegetables that contain high levels of fiber are sweet potatoes, salad greens, raisins, apples, rhubarb, bananas, and prunes. Make sure that you are incorporating these types of fruits and vegetables each day to insure the reoccurrence of constipation and also to prevent even the onset of constipation.

Useful Treatment Tips

> ➤ Castor oil is also a very effective and popular natural laxative. Simply take one teaspoon of castor

oil in the early mornings will help with clearing your digestive track as well as cleaning your whole digestive system.

➢ Orange juice and olive oil can also work hand in hand to curing your constipation. Simply mix half of a cup of orange juice and 1-2 tablespoons of olive oil and you will find constipation no longer a concern of yours. You can repeat this mixture twice a day for best results.

➢ Aloe Vera is also a very helpful remedy for curing constipation. Aloe Vera not only comes in gel form but in juice form also. Aloe Vera juice can dramatically ease your pain and discomfort due to constipation. Having some Aloe Vera juice in the mornings and then again in the evening times will help loosen up your digestive track and cleanse your whole digestive system.

➢ You can also mix a quarter of a cup of carrot juice, a half of a cup of sauerkraut juice, and one cup of tomato juice and create a cocktail for instant constipation relief. For best results consume this mixture up to three times a day.

Depression

Depression is a very serious illness that affects many people worldwide. There are many methods to treating depression whether it is through counseling, prescriptions for depression medication, changes in your daily routine or rituals, changing your diet, etc. However, there can be a better and more natural way to treat your depression without those nasty side effects. Here are a few natural home remedies to help treat your depression and give a better mood level. Note: Depression is a serious and very dangerous illness and professional help is required, these are only home remedies that can help teat common symptoms of depression.

Caffeine – can help give you the boost you need to start your everyday activities. Although some studies have shown that large amounts of caffeine-intake can increase the rate of depression. However, as long as you are only consuming 1 or 2 cups per day to help keep your symptoms at ease, then you will not produce this effect. You can also try switching from coffee to green tea. Green tea only has half of the amount of caffeine that is found in normal caffeinated drinks and also provides you with tons of nutritional benefits.

Deep Sea Cold Water Fish – Trying incorporating deep sea cold water fish to your diet regularly. One of the most important nutrients, Omega 3, is very beneficial when trying to lift up your spirits and your mood level. Studies have shown that consuming foods that contain high amounts of omega 3 has been proven to lifting your mood. Deep sea cold water fish that have the highest levels of omega 3 are sardines, mackerel, and salmon.

Chocolate – I think most people would be surprised to see chocolate as a home remedy for depression. Although it sounds too good to be true, it is. However, there are details as to what types of chocolate actually uplift your mood. Studies have shown that eating dark chocolate is actually the source that will most effectively contribute to changing your mood for the better. Although many prefer the lighter chocolate than dark chocolate, due to its more bitter taste, the lighter chocolate has no affect what so ever in your mood. You can also find organic bitter chocolate at your finer health food stores and have been proven to also lift your spirits and your symptoms of depression.

Home-made Infusions - Preparing this little home remedy can be a very tasty one also. To create this concoction you boil a teaspoon of holy basil or Indian basil and a half of a teaspoon of sage per cup of tea. By drinking this infusion at least twice a day you will see your mood and energy increase dramatically. You can also alternatively powder the seeds of one to two green cardamoms and then add this to a cup of boiling water and a little bit of sugar. You will also want to consume this infusion up to two times a day for best results.

Herbal Treatments – There are many herbal treatments that have also been studied and proven to help depression related symptoms. All of the herbs can each be added to a brew of your favorite herbal tea and be created into a infusion drink. Lemon balm is most commonly used to help calm a person's physical tension. The herb Skullcap can also be used in herbal treatment for depression by easing panic attacks and the number of occurrences. Indian Ginseng, or ashwaganha, is an herb that has been used for hundreds of thousands of years in India. Indian Ginseng not only helps reduce your stress but also calms your entire nervous system. It also helps with calmness, as well as helps keep away any negative thoughts from running through your head. This natural pure herb not only nourishes your brain but also helps in brain functioning better as well as more effectively.

Bacopa, or brahmi, is also another herb that has been tested and proven to help with depression symptoms. This herb gives your brain the soothing effect that it looks for when battling depression. Not only does it cure your brain of unwanted anxieties but it also helps improve your memory. Sumenta is normally found as a herbal supplement that combines adaptogenic, anxiolytics, and anti-stress ingredients and can be found in many nutritional and health stores. For many people that deal with depression also deal with anxiety and using this herbal supplement you can kill two birds with one stone. One of the most popular and most well-known herbal treatments in aiding depression related symptoms is St. John's Wart. This is also a natural herb and is used as a mood stabilizer and also helps in aiding to fight against depression as well as anxiety spells. You can also find this herb at your local pharmacy or nutritional store.

Useful Treatment Tips

> Eating an apple with some milk and honey can also act as a mood lifter and helps reduce your symptoms of depression.

> Try incorporating almonds into your diet. Chewing anywhere from 10-15 almonds daily is very beneficial to your mood and brain levels. However, they are found most effective is they have been soaked overnight and eaten the next morning.

> You can also boil a cup of water and add a few rose petals and some sugar also and have a great mixture to help soothe your depression symptoms, mainly your depressed feeling.

> You can also try incorporating a few drops of aromatic herbal oils in your bath water and take a much needed hour long bath which will not only relieve some stress but ease your mind and your thought patterns. This is also a good way to calm and soothe your body giving off those good endorphins.

> Root of asparagus is another widely used treatment option when it comes to easing depression symptoms. You can take 1-2 grams of powdered root once daily.

> Cashew nuts are very rich in Thiamine and Vitamin B. Chewing cashews not only stimulates your

nervous system but also helps with symptoms of depression.

Earache

I am pretty sure that most everybody has had an earache at least one time in their life and you know as well as I do they can be a very painful, uncomfortable, and irritable condition to have. Earaches can make it very hard to sleep, can take on associated symptoms such as headaches, swollen jaws, and even vomiting. Adults most commonly acquire an earache through swimmer's ear but for babies and small children they can acquire an earache quite often. However, earaches can also be a sign of an infection somewhere else in your body, so be sure to check in with your regular physician if your earache accompanies a fever or persists for more than 3-4 days. Here are of the top natural home remedies that you can try that will help you with the pain of an earache as well as treatment and prevention from an earache.

Useful Treatment Tips

> ➢ Take one to two teaspoons of chamomile flowers and place them in a pain with one cup of water. Boil and steep the flowers for around 10-15 minutes. After you have steeped the chamomile flowers in the boiling water strain the water and place the hot flowers in a cloth and place it on the ear that is sore. Leave the cloth on the ear for 15-20 minutes at a time. You will soon find that your earache is in the works of clearing up in little to no time.

➢ You can also try taking peeling 2 cloves of garlic and then mixing the cut up cloves with two teaspoons of mustard oil. You then heat the mixture until the garlic turns black. Remove from heat and strain and allow the mixture to cool until it is lukewarm. You then apply 3-4 drops into the ear using a cotton swab or dropper. This can help with many of the symptoms associated with an earache, mostly with the pain you receive due to an earache.

➢ By mixing some garlic oil with around 3 drops of grape seed extract and then dropping the mixture into the affected ear. This is a tested and proven way to alleviate a ton of earache pain.

➢ You can also try taking a few whole basil leaves and then grind them into a blender or juicer to make it into a juice. Then you will want to place two drops of the basil leaf juice inside the affected ear. This is a major pain reducer and also helps with the reduction of fever. You can also try this with the juice of garlic. After blending garlic cloves in a blender or juicer you will take several drops of the garlic juice in a dropper and place the mixture in the affected ear. This is also great for pain and also works as a natural antibiotic and has been tested and proven to be extremely effective towards earaches that are caused by an infection in the ear.

➢ You can also try placing a few drops of warm olive oil, tea tree oil, mineral oil, or sweet oil into the ear that is infected or aching. These specific oils can most commonly be found in your local pharmacy or health and nutritional stores and have been used for ages for the relief of earache pain.

➤ You may also want to try taking one teaspoon of sesame oil and adding a clove of garlic to the oil. You will then want to heat up the mixture until the mixture becomes lukewarm. You will then want to place anywhere from 3-4 drops of the mixture into the ear that has the earache and then lie on your side for around 10-15 minutes

➤ Take 1-2 tablespoons of mustard oil and place in a pan. Take a small radish and chop it into small-medium pieces. Add the chopped radish to the mustard oil and warm the mixture gently. Then place a couple of drops of the mixture into the affected ear. This can help majorly with your earache pain.

➤ You can also warm the leaves of a mango in a small amount of water. You then take the juice from the mango leaves and place a few drops into the affected ear. This will help with the pain and discomfort associated with your earache also.

➤ Another old home remedy that has been used for many years is by taking a capful of hydrogen peroxide and places it into the affected ear. The ear will fizz and bubble, this is normal. Peroxide is really good for clearing up any infections and allows the ear to dry out. You can also mix the peroxide half and half with water. Make sure to let the ear drain after applying the peroxide.

➤ You may also want try cutting up a piece of garlic and wrapping it with a piece of a cotton ball. Then immerse the cotton ball with alcohol. You will then squeeze the excess alcohol and put it in the ear that is hurting. This is a very effective home remedy that will clear the pain and discomfort due to an earache.

➤ You can also try to immerse a half of a cotton ball in olive oil. Then place the cotton ball in the microwave for around 15-20 seconds until the cotton ball is warm, not hot. You will then squeeze out the excess oil from the cotton ball so that the cotton ball is dampened by the oil. Place the cotton ball in the affected ear and let it stay in for around 15-20 minutes. You can repeat this procedure continuously throughout the day for your earache and to help with pain.

Gout

Gout can be a very painful condition for anyone to have and for most people even prescriptions that they get from their doctor isn't enough to cure the pain. Gout is a type of metabolic arthritis and for a lot of people can put a strain and a painful constant reminder to everyday life activities. However, many people with gout have found that home remedies have become more reliable to use than any doctor's prescription and relieves their aches and pains due to gout. Here are a few home remedies that you can try to help your pain as well as your frustration to gout.

Cherries and Cherry Juice – Cherries are a great home remedy to help neutralize the uric acid that causes gout. Cherries are also very high in magnesium and vitamin C, which are two minerals that not only promote circulation but also help in digestion. You can consume cherries in virtually any form such as canned cherries, dried cherries, fresh fruit cherries, sweet yellow cherries, black cherries, and cherry juice and all forms have been proven to dramatically prevent gout attacks as well as helps eliminate inflammation during a gout attack. Through a recent study, people who ate a half pound of cherries were shown to lower their uric acid levels down to the normal range in every person they studied. Although this does seem like a lot of cherries to consume, I am sure that many people would choose that alternative rather than deal with the aches and pains that gout causes them. Eating at least 10 cherries daily or consuming at least 16 ounces of cherry juice 1-2 times daily has been proven to be standard guidelines to prevent gout flare-ups. Keep in mind, that although cherries have no known side effects, eating too much of one food can cause you some major stomach distress such as constipation or diarrhea. Therefore, while you should consume the above guidelines for cherries and cherry juice, you should also ingest the amount that your body is comfortable with also.

Water – water plays a big factor in the reduction of uric acid in your body and also eliminates it from your system at a much faster rate. Not only is water safe and natural to drink and is also side effect free, but also drinking plenty of it daily helps in proper digestion. You can also add a high PH to your water such as alko-pro, can also help neutralize the acids in your body. You can also try using chlorella, wheatgrass, and spirulina which all help in the alkalinizing of the body. This also works the same way as drinking high PH water levels. Consuming at least 2-3 liters of water per day is an efficient amount to flush your whole system clean. Keep in mind that it is important to lower your intake of beverages that cause dehydration such as caffeinated and alcoholic drinks. You will want to stick to hydrating drinks such as water, herbal tea, and fruit juice.

Charcoal – I know it sounds crazy to even use charcoal besides in your grill, however charcoal has become one of the top home remedies for relieving gout pains for a person. Using activated charcoal poultice has been studied and shown to dramatically reduce inflammation as well as helps eliminate uric acid. Simply mix a half of a cup of activated powdered charcoal with 3-7 tablespoons of ground flaxseed. Once the mixture becomes mealy, warm water can then be added to turn this mixture into a paste. The paste is then placed on the joint that is inflamed and covered with a cloth or plastic dressing. You will have to change your dressings periodically every 4 hours and can be left on overnight. Keep in mind that charcoal poultice will stain virtually any fabric that it touches, so handle with care when using this home remedy to help ease your pains with gout.

Low Purine Diet – along with home remedies you will also want to control your diet by eliminating foods that are high in purines, which are not only known to trigger gout attacks but can also worsen gout attacks also. Studies have shown, that half of the uric acid produced by your body is a result of purine rich foods consumed in a person's diet. Foods that are high in purine and that should be avoided are wild game, sardines, scallops, mackerel, organ meats, meat extract, gravies, and sweetbreads. Focusing your diet more towards vegetable protein, dairy products, and increased water intake, is a great diet plan that should be followed to show an effective decrease in purine as well as prevents sudden painful gout attacks. However, you will want to keep in mind that some foods that are high in purines contain certain essential nutrients that your body requires such as protein. So make sure that even though you are trying to eliminate purine in your system, that you also replace them so that your body is receiving the adequate nutrients to stay healthy.

Juniper Oil and Devil's Claw – Both juniper oil and devil's claw can dramatically reduce the inflammation due to gout. Taking just a few drops of juniper oil and making a compress to the affected area is the remedy to easing pain in your joints due to gout. Juniper oil will also help break down toxic deposits. You can also help speed your recovery by consuming water which will wash the deposits out of your system. Devil's claw is also another anti-inflammatory herb that helps ease the pain of gout. You will need to keep in mind that you do not need to take this herb if you have diabetes or are taking a blood thinning medication. As an added extra bonus, devil's claw also helps reduce uric acid buildup. You can find devil's claw at your local nutritional store and other stores that sell herbal remedies.

Garlic and Thyme – Garlic is used by many people to cure tones of conditions that harp their everyday lives. Gout is no different when it comes to what wonders garlic can do for you. Garlic actually inhibits the production of uric acid which is the source to gout attacks and inflammation. Using garlic in raw, powdered, and pill form are all very effective ways to consume garlic in your diet and dramatically help all of your gout symptoms. Thyme is also a great source to reducing uric acid in your body. Thyme has been used since the 1600's for the relief of gout pain, first used by people of high royalty. Using thyme in your herbal tea will show you immediate anti-inflammatory properties that are formed by gout.

Hot and Cold Compressions – Applying hot and cold compressions to the affected area can also aid in the relief of gout pain caused by inflammation. This helps to increase the blood circulation and in doing so you can reduce inflammation and relieve gout pain. The common method to using hot and cold compressions is by using heat for 3 minutes, and then cold for 30 seconds. Continue to repeat this process but make sure than you do this for no more than 20 minutes and always remember to finish with the cold compressions. Although this is not a permanent solution for your gout pain, it can however make a dramatic relief to the symptoms associated with gout.

Useful Treatment Tips

➤ You can also use baking soda as a cure for gout. However, you will want to check with your doctor to make sure that this is a home remedy that you can try because of the high levels of sodium in baking soda that is involved. Using a half of a teaspoon of baking soda powder in a glass of water before you go to sleep and first thing when you get up can provide you with pain and inflammatory relief. Make sure that you don't exceed more than 3 teaspoons a day. Make sure that when you purchase baking soda that you get aluminum free baking soda for the best effects on uric acid levels.

➤ You can also soak the affected area in warm water with some muscle relaxing soap or salts to help soothe the area and help with pain also. Try using

Epsom salt that contains magnesium. Raising your magnesium levels may improve your heart and circulation as well as also lowers your blood pressure. The Epson salt will help flush away the toxins and heavy metals that are present in your body. Simply add two cups of Epsom salt to warm water as the bathtub fills. Stay in the bath until the water starts losing its heat. This is a major remedy that can dramatically decrease your symptoms associated with gout.

➢ Consuming fresh strawberries also helps in neutralizing uric acid. Strawberries contain high concentrations of Vitamin C as well as fruit acids and minerals such as potassium, calcium, iron, magnesium zinc, and manganese, all of which aid in the reduction of uric acid.

➢ Apple Cider Vinegar is also a great remedy to use and is used by many old-timers. This is a remedy that has been used for centuries in the cure of a lot of common conditions, such as gout. Try using 2 tablespoons of organic apple cider vinegar and mix it with 2 tablespoons of organic honey at least two times a day and within a few hours of the onset of your pain from gout, your pain will start to subside.

➢ Using high doses of vitamin C has also been proven to reduce uric acid levels. You can go to your local nutritional store or your pharmacy and get non-acidic vitamin C supplements and take one tablet two times a day. Make sure that the supplement pills are 1,000mg because this is the most effective dosing for gout when consuming vitamin C supplements and has shown to be more powerful towards your pains associated with gout.

Hangover

Many people suffer from a hangover after a fun night on the town. This leaves them wishing they had never touched it in the first place. The symptoms associated with a hangover include excruciating pain in your head, almost like a classic migraine. Many people look for the perfect home remedies to treat their symptoms of a hangover. Here are the most popular and most commonly used home remedies for a hangover.

Vitamin C – is a very effective way to get rid of a hangover very quickly. Drinking lots of orange juice or any other citrus drink is the best way to recover from a hangover. Your body will have dehydrated due to the alcohol consumption the night before and vitamin C is the key to rehydrating yourself.

Honey – is also a good home remedy for hangover symptoms. Honey is very high in fructose which is beneficial in breaking down alcohol. Brewing hot tea flavored with lime juice and then sweetened with honey can dramatically help your hangover symptoms. You can also consume a few tablespoons of honey the morning of your hangover and you will also receive relief from hangover symptoms as well. You do not want to use sugar because sugar contains sucrose which can absorb the fructose. Definitely a no-no if you want your hangover symptoms to be relieved.

Bananas and Apples – are also very effective in curing hangover symptoms. These fruits naturally restore your body back to normal. Bananas are a very effective home remedy because when a person drinks alcohol they have frequent urination, which only drains the body of potassium. As we all know bananas are very rich in potassium and will dramatically restore your potassium levels back to normal. Eating an apple is also very beneficial and can also relieve symptoms of a hangover.

Ginger – is also another home remedy that can be used to help aid your aching hangover. Ginger naturally soothes the liner in your stomach and also alleviates any nausea that you might be having. Simply boil slices of fresh ginger root in approximately 4 cups of water for around 10-15 minutes. You then strain the ginger and then add the juice from one fresh orange as well as the juice from a half of a lemon. You can also add a half of a cup of honey which will double your dose of a hangover symptom killer. Consuming ginger ale can also give you the same benefits. Drink at least 8 ounces of ginger ale early in the morning and you will find your hangover symptoms diminish to nothing.

Consuming Food – Although food is probably the last thing on your mind, it can be the best thing for you and your hangover symptoms. Try eating a bowl of chicken broth and some plain toast. This will absorb any alcohol left over in your system and the chicken broth has properties to help get the body in balance and back to normal. You can also try a small bowl or rice as it has high properties to defeat nausea as well as absorbs liquids very quickly.

Gatorade or PowerAde – This home remedy is a simple and easy remedy to help ease your hangover symptoms. Gatorade and PowerAde are packed with loads of nutrients and can help resupply your electrolytes. When you consume alcohol your body is instantly dehydrated and a great way to rehydrate your body is by consuming these types of drinks. These types of drinks also have properties to help give you energy. If you have ever had a hangover you know that you feel very tired and weak. Consuming Gatorade or PowerAde can aid in making you feel replenished and at the same time alleviates your hangover symptoms in little to no time at all.

Ice Compressions – Normally the biggest symptom associated with a hangover is a crushing headache. This can easily be cured by applying ice cold compresses. Simply place some crushed ice into a plastic bag. Wrap the plastic bag around your head with a towel. You will want to make sure that you are applying the ice in the throbbing areas of your skull. You can also soak a wash cloth in cold water and then drape it over your forehead or simply lay back (which is more than likely what you would prefer to be doing anyways). Leave the ice cold compressions on for 15-20 minutes. Repeat the process periodically until your headache diminishes.

"Hair of the Dog" – this is a very well-known and common home remedy that is used to cure a hangover. This is a home remedy that has been used for many years and actually has been proven to work. In this home remedy, although it might sound crazy, you will want to consume 1 alcoholic beverage, preferably a canned beer. The trick is to only consume 1 alcoholic beverage and your hangover symptoms will clear.

Coffee and Pickle Juice – Both coffee and pickle juice have been proven to cure hangover symptoms. However, when it comes to coffee you will want to make sure that you don't add any sugar to it. Instead flavor your coffee with honey which also helps in the aid of a hangover. Due to the vinegar in pickle juice this is also a great home remedy for a hangover. The vinegar in the pickle juice helps to flush out your blood stream. This means alleviating any presence of alcohol.

Water – as simple as it may sound water is a great remedy for curing a hangover. Like I said before hangovers are due to dehydration of the body so it is very important that you drink plenty of water to rehydrate yourself and also flush out the toxins in your system due to the alcohol. Drink a few glasses of water before going to bed as well as when you wake up. Drinking water before you go to bed will help dramatically because your body will be flushing itself while you are resting. Make sure to consume at least 8-10 glasses of water the day of the hangover to help replenish your body and get your levels back in the normal range.

Raw Cabbage –can also be used as a home remedy for treating a hangover. Simply chew up pieces of raw cabbage to gain instant relief from a headache. Try doing this periodically during the day because it also has properties to help with energy. Using tomato juice and cabbage together can create a duo against symptoms of hangovers.

High Blood Pressure

High blood pressure or hypertension is a very common health condition that many people deal with each and every day. High blood pressure can be a very serious condition as, the risk of stroke and heart attack are increased greatly for people with high blood pressure. Lowering your high blood pressure is very hard and most commonly people with high blood pressure end up getting a prescription from their physician for this condition. You can however skip the prescription and reduce your blood pressure the natural way with these common home remedies.

Garlic – not only lowers your blood pressure but also relaxes your blood vessels which means that your blood vessels will not tighten up. Garlic can also help lower your risk for heart disease. You can take garlic in either raw form or by pill form; both are very effective in lowering your blood pressure. This home remedy has been clinically tested and proven to lower a person's blood pressure greatly!

Fish Oil – Although fish oil doesn't directly lower your blood pressure, it does however work to keep your entire circulatory system as well as your heart in tip top shape. Remember that the first step to lowering your high blood pressure is by improving the areas that are causing the condition. Fish from the deep blue sea also contain omega-3 fatty acids such as tuna. You can find pills forms of omega-3, however the best and most effective way to benefit from it is by eating it raw. Grilling and broiling these types of fish can also help with lowering your blood pressure. Try adding spices as well to the fish that you are cooking, certain spices also help lower blood pressure and will make your fish tastier.

Bananas, Broccoli, and Celery – Bananas have been proven to reduce your blood pressure greatly. This is because bananas are rich and high in potassium and through clinical studies has proven to dramatically reduce your blood pressure. Bananas and foods high in potassium can reduce your blood pressure up to 20 points. You can also try other foods that are high in potassium such as avocados, prunes, raisins, and dried apricots.

A high fiber diet has also shown to greatly lower a person's blood pressure. Broccoli is very high in fiber and has been proven to lower your blood pressure also. If you don't particularly like broccoli there are many other foods that you can consume that are high in fiber such as Brussels sprouts, cabbage, carrots, mushrooms, peppers, spinach, and sweet potatoes.

Celery is also a very good antidote to lowering your blood pressure naturally. This is because celery contains 3-N-butylphthalide, which is a phytochemical that is found in celery. This particular property has been tested, studied, and found to lower your blood pressure. Celery has also been proven to greatly reduce your stress hormones which constrict your blood vessels, something you definitely don't want your blood vessels to do when you have high blood pressure... this will only raise your blood pressure. You can also try celery in soup form and has been proven to work just as well as eating a celery stalk.

Magnesium – Magnesium can also help in lowering your blood pressure. Magnesium can be found in your bones, organs, and body tissue and is a micronutrient. Magnesium and potassium work hand in hand which is why magnesium aids in reducing your blood pressure. Foods that are high in magnesium are shrimp, tofu, salmon spinach, bananas, rice, and sardines. Magnesium can also be found in a pill form over the counter and can also be very effect, although daily consumption of foods containing magnesium is proved to drop your blood pressure more quickly and effectively. For best results consume around 400 milligrams a day of magnesium and watch your high blood pressure decrease more and more each day.

Useful Treatment Tips

> Grapefruits and lemons are also very beneficial in the treatment of your high blood pressure. This is because both fruits contain Vitamin P which is effective in preventing capillary fragility and also tones up your arteries.

> Indian gooseberry juice and honey can also help you lower your blood pressure when you mix the two ingredients together. Try taking two tablespoons of Indian gooseberry juice and honey mixed together. You can take this mixture every morning on an empty stomach and can be the

perfect antidote to naturally lower your blood pressure without the hassle of taking a pill.

➢ Try consuming at least two to three cloves of garlic twice daily. This will not only lower your blood pressure but it also restricts the spasms of small arteries and also moderates your heart beat as well as your pulse rate.

➢ You can also try making a parsley leaf beverage by simmering 20 grams of fresh parsley leaves in 250 ml of water. You can drink this mixture frequently throughout the day and helps improve arterial health.

➢ Using one teaspoon of fenugreek seeds with water each morning on an empty stomach can also maintain and control your blood pressure throughout the day.

➢ You can also mix one teaspoon of cayenne pepper with a half of a cup of lukewarm water daily. This is also a very effective home remedy that will lower your blood pressure dramatically.

Knee Pain

Knee pain can be very common among elderly people, athletes, small children with growing pains, as well as people that workout. Knee pain can not only impair your mobility but also puts a strain on a number of different areas of the body such as your back, neck, and even your feet. Although you shouldn't have persistent knew pain and if your symptoms don't clear up within a week, you should probably consult a physician. However, there are some home remedies that can help you with everyday common knee pain and arthritis in your knee. Here are a few of the top home remedies that can help your aching knees and provide you with the relief you are looking for.

Rest – Everyone should know that with any kind of muscle or joint pain that the best thing for your body in general is rest. This also holds true when it comes to knee pain. Rest has to be the most simple and a very effective way to alleviate any kind of knee pain. You will first want to lay in a comfortable position where your knees are relaxed. You will want to place them in a normal position without any bending. This method not only creates a way for your blood to flow naturally and moves with ease but also helps in the circulation of your whole body. Staying off of your feet for long periods of time will allow the muscles around your knees to relax and recover from the strain that has been placed on your knees.

Cold Compresses – If you endure knee pain due to an injury such as a fall or a sports injury then you might find that cold compresses on your injured knee can make a worlds difference on the pain you are having. In this method you will want to apply ice to the knee in intervals of 20 minutes for up to three times a day. Keep a close eye on the skin also while you follow this method. Cold compresses can be a way for you to give your knee pain from an injury immediate relief.

Knee Braces – Knee braces can become an athlete's best friend when it comes to knee pain due to a sports injury. However, knee braces are also used among elders and people that have a lot of strenuous activities that involve the bending of their knees. Knee braces give your knees the proper support as well as helps with knee mobility. Most commonly athletes that use knee braces not only wear them off the field but also on the field to help from further injury. Keep in mind, a small injury can turn into a big injury in little to know time without proper treatment.

Elevation – This is another method that can provide anyone with knee pain a little bit of relief for their sore knees. It is always a good thing to elevate your leg when you have knee pain or if you have acquired a knee injury. You will want to make sure that you are elevating your knee at a heart level. This will help dramatically in the decrease of inflammation that could be attribute to your knee pain. You can also place pillows stacked up to raise your legs providing instant relief and circulation to your knees and body in general.

Omega 3 – Omega 3 fatty acids are very essential when it comes to mending those damaged joints. Try incorporating a little sweet water fish in your diet weekly to alleviate common knee pains. Salt water seafood includes tuna, herring, sardines, and salmon, which are all very rich in omega 3 fatty acids. You can also consume healthy fresh vegetables such broccoli, carrots, and spinach, as well as fruits such as pineapple, grapes, and bananas. Also, flavonoid rich food items provide a benefit to treating a knee pain due to a knee injury.

Yoga, Posture, and Daily Exercise – You can also try your hand at some yoga if you experience several bouts of knee pain. Doing yoga regularly along with breathing exercises helps you to relax and can also cure knee aches because believe it or not some pains are caused by mental stress. Yoga can also provide your knee with increased flexibility which means a decrease in strains or pulled muscles associated with the knee. The best part about yoga is all of the relief given to your knee and joint are being performed in an all-natural way.

Posture also has a lot to do with many common joint and muscle pains. A special technique that helps improve your posture while providing you with pain relief is called the warrior posture method. You can perform this method by standing with your feet 4 foot apart, you then turn your left foot in an inward direction and your right foot in an outward direction. You will want to keep your chest facing straight and in front of your body. You will then stretch out both of your arms and bend them in the direction of your right knee and turn your head to look at your right knee. You can repeat this process with each leg and can provide you with a better stretched out knee and will strengthen your knees for less knee injuries due to strains or pulled muscles.

Useful Treatment Tips

> ➤ You can also try to walk with the support of a cane that can serve as very effective relief to any type of knee pain. This can prove to be very beneficial for those who suffer from arthritis in their knee. Keep in mind that when using a cane you will want to support the cane in the hand that is opposite to the knee with the pain.

> ➤ Green tea is very rich in antioxidants that have bone boosting properties. Studies have also shown that green tea may be used as a pain reliever.

> ➤ Cortisone injections for mild arthritis and Gold injection and methotrexate for rheumatoid arthritis are used a lot of the times for suppressing knee joint pain.

> ➤ Glucosamine supplements are also very capable of restoring and rebuilding cartilages, therefore making this a helpful supplement for continuous knee pain.

Poison Ivy

Poison Ivy is a very common condition that people acquire when they get close to a poison ivy plant. Poison Ivy contains urushiol, which the plant uses to protect itself from foraging animals. However, urushiol is very harmful to humans and is a skin irritant. Some people may not be affected by poison ivy even if they are in direct contact while others can just look at poison ivy and contract the irritating and itchy rashes associated with poison ivy. For those who you who are blessed with the ability to contract poison ivy... have no fear, there are some natural home remedies that can help your poison ivy symptoms and also treat the skin condition as well. Here are the top home remedies for poison ivy.

Oatmeal – is a very common home remedy used to help with the treatment and helps with the symptoms of poison ivy. The oatmeal provides not only the soothing sensation to the affected area or areas but also leaves a white powdery finish that helps dry out the poison ivy rashes and speeds up the treatment rate. You can use oatmeal in two different ways, an oatmeal bath or applying an oatmeal paste to the affected area or areas. Use the bath method, simply pour a whole box of oatmeal into warm bathwater and soak in the bath for at least 20-30 minutes. Make sure that when you get out of the bathtub that you do not dry yourself off, leaving the powdery residue will help dry out the rashes more quickly. You can also try the other method by applying oatmeal directly to the rashes. In this method you will want to mix 3 cups of oats is a bowl of boiling water. The oatmeal and water will create a paste like consistency. When the paste is warm enough to tolerate, apply the paste to the affected areas. You can also add 1-2 tablespoons of baking soda to also help with itching. Using the oatmeal home remedy provides you with instant relief from itching almost immediately.

Baking Soda – This is a classic and commonly used home remedy to help with the symptoms of poison ivy as well as helps treat poison ivy outbreaks also. Like the oatmeal, you can form a paste out of baking soda and then apply it to the affected area or areas. Take three teaspoons of baking soda and mix it with one teaspoons of clean sterile water. This will form a thick paste. Apply the paste to the rashes and allow the paste to dry. This helps treat the watery blisters and also helps alleviate the itching sensation.

Goldenseal – Another home remedy that you can try to treat your poison ivy is by using a skin wash with Goldenseal. In this home remedy you will need to mix a tablespoon of powdered goldenseal root with a cup of lukewarm to hot water. This will make a paste similar to oatmeal and baking soda. After the mixture cools down apply the goldenseal treatment to all of the affected areas. This herb has anti-inflammatory properties and also rapidly dries up the poison ivy blisters and rashes. Note that this home remedy can also be used in cases of poison oak and can provide instant itching relief.

Salt and Aloe Vera – This is a home remedy that has been used for many years and has been proved to be very effective in the treatment of poison ivy. There are however a couple of steps to go by when performing this home remedy. You will first want to wash the affected area or areas with rubbing alcohol and then wash the area with soap and warm water. Then you will pour plain table salt onto all of the affected areas and leave it on the rashes for 5-10 minutes. The salt not only will help to reduce the chances of the poison ivy spreading but also helps with any other further infections as well as helps with itching relief also. After you have let the salt stand on the rashes you will then then wash off the salt from the affected areas and apply a heavy coat of Aloe Vera onto the rashes. This will provide you with immediate cooling as well as provides you with instant relief to itching and also to any burning sensations.

Banana Peels - This is another home remedy that has been tested and proven to provide you with instant itching relief. Simply take the peels from a banana and rub the inner side of the peel of the banana over the affected area or areas. You will be surprised in the instant and immediate relief you receive by using this home remedy.

Vitamins – Vitamin C and E help dramatically in the treatment of poison ivy. Both Vitamin C and Vitamin E can be taken in large doses and acts as a detoxifier and an antihistamine. What you will want to do in this home remedy is dissolve a Vitamin C or E tablet in warm water and then washing the affected areas. By squeezing the juice from a lemon or orange is also an effective wash to use. Just simply dabbing the mixture on the affected areas does the trick also.

Useful Treatment Tips

➤ You may also want to try applying garlic oil or olive oil. Both oils can dry out rashes as well as provide relief to your itching symptoms.

➤ Washing the affected areas with running water can also help in the skin itching and will also help wash away histamines.

➤ Apple cider vinegar and white vinegar also helps draw out poison ivy and also gives relief to poison ivy symptoms. Apply both vinegars directly to all affected rashes and immediate itching relief and treatment will start.

Psoriasis

Psoriasis is a very common skin disorder and is cause by faulty metabolic functions or a drop in the body's immunity system. This skin disorder affects both sexes and race and is commonly found in people between the ages of 15-30 years old. With psoriasis the skin becomes thick and then develops red, silvery patches that resemble scales and leaves people with this skin disorder with constant itching and pain. Psoriasis mainly affects elbows, scalp, knees, the skin behind the ears, and the trunk. Although this is not a contagious skin disorder it still leaves it's recipients with pain, irritation, and inflammation. However, there are some home remedies that you can try to ease the symptoms that psoriasis causes.

Oatmeal – has been tested and proven to help with the symptoms associated with psoriasis. However, the types of oats that you will have to use are not your everyday oats that you use to make your favorite oatmeal for breakfast. The kind of oatmeal that you will have to use is powdered oatmeal, which you can make yourself with the use of a blender. What you will do is simply take a few handfuls of the powdered oatmeal into a bath filled with lukewarm running water. Since the powdered oatmeal is so fine, it will almost instantly start turning into a milky, slimy consistency. When you start your oatmeal bath make sure that the water is still lukewarm and stay in the water for around 30-45 minutes. Not only will the oatmeal bath bend to the skin but it will also help keep your skin moisturized as well as reduces the soreness and redness all in this one method. This method will help your psoriasis condition so much that you won't look at oatmeal as just a breakfast meal again, but as a natural and beneficial method to easing your psoriasis pain.

Licorice – Although many people cringe at even the taste of licorice, you won't have to worry about eating any licorice for this method. Licorice is an old remedy that has been used for many years and it doesn't have to be ingested as the sole source to helping psoriasis symptoms is by external application to the affected areas that hold the psoriasis patches. Licorice is useful in the treatment of psoriasis do to it containing the compound called glycyrrhetinic acid, which is present in the veiny stems of the licorice. The compound that is found in the licorice stem has anti-inflammatory properties which helps with the soreness and redness that psoriasis causes. In this treatment option you can do one of two different methods, get licorice root and boil it down until the water is evaporated or you can just as easily use some concentrated licorice tincture that is available at your local pharmacy or nutritional store. What you will need to do is drip around 3-4 drops onto a cotton ball of sterile gauze and then apply it directly to the skin where the psoriasis patches are found.

Chamomile – This is another old remedy for psoriasis that had been used by many people and first originated in Europe. This particular plant contains the compounds called flavonoids, which has been tested and proven to have anti-inflammatory properties, which is why this is a great method for treating psoriasis. However, make sure then when using this method of treatment that you don't have hay fever at the time of consuming chamomile. Chamomile is a part of the ragweed family and because of that it produces tons of pollen. The best and most effective way to use this treatment method is as compressions or body dressing. What you will need to do is to take a handful of chamomile flowers and one cup of hot water and wait for the flower to welt; this process takes around 25-30 minutes. After that process is complete you will want to strain the flowers out and soak a clean towel in the water and chamomile mixture. After you have soaked up the mixture in the clean town you then wrap the towel around the affected areas. This is a great and simply way to cure your psoriasis symptoms.

Aloe Vera – This is a very good herb and the gel that you get out of the Aloe Vera plant has tons of benefits. You simply apply Aloe Vera gel, either in raw form or processed over the affected areas. You can also take Aloe Vera gel and combine it with a vitamin E solution and apply the mixture of the two to the psoriasis patches. You can also mix it with turmeric powder and create a powerful concoction also. Make sure to check with your doctor before applying this to your skin because the FDA has not yet approved this treatment for psoriasis symptoms.

Useful Treatment Tips

> You can try taking 4 marigold flower heads and boil them in approximately 4 cups of water for two minutes and then let the mixture coo. Massaging this mixture on the affected areas and then washing it off with a mild soap will reduce skin irritation due

to psoriasis symptoms. A few drops of lemon juice or cider vinegar can also be added to the rinsing water for a better wash.

➤ Hot Epsom salt baths also are widely used for the treatment of psoriasis. In this method the skin absorbs the salt and in return improves your blood circulation. Another great tip is after bathing applying olive oil also gives you better results to your psoriasis symptoms.

➤ You may also want to try 1 drop of oregano oil and 2 drops of calendula oil mixed together in one cup of olive oil. After you have made up the mixture you then apply the mixture to the affected area.

➤ De-veined cabbage leaves can also be applied to the area that is affected by psoriasis and can relieve the symptoms dramatically.

➤ You may also want to make sure to take regular sea bathing or you can simply apply sea water onto the areas of skin that need to be treated and not only will you find a dramatic difference in the symptoms but also less of an occurrence.

➤ You can also try a mixture of Aloe Vera gel and olive oil. Simply mix the two together and then apply this to the affected area. The Aloe Vera will help with the pain of psoriasis and the olive oil acts as a moisturizer preventing the skin from drying out and becoming itchy.

Ringworm

Ringworm is a fungal infection that can affect almost anyone who comes in contact with it. You can contract ringworm on literally any part of your body and they can also be very hard to get rid of and can take up to 4 weeks to completely go away. However more and more people have found that using home remedies to clear up the fungal infection is more effective than even prescription medication. Here are some of the most popular home remedies to treat ringworm.

Athlete's Foot Spray – this is a very commonly known home remedy to clear up ringworm. You can get athlete's foot spray at any sporting goods store or your local pharmacy. Simply spray the athlete's foot spray on the affected area. You can do this procedure often and should be performed on a daily basis until the ringworm has completely cleared. You can also bandage the ringworm to make sure that you do not pass it to anyone else but you also want to make sure to let it air out also. Athlete's foot spray contains properties to kill and fight against fungal infections including ringworm. You will find that this will clear the ringworm up very quickly and in little to no time you will be rid of the ringworm completely.

Holy Basil – Another great home remedy that has been used for many years is using holy basil to treat ringworm. Simply extract the juice from the leaves of basil and then apply it to the area of skin that has the ringworm. Keep applying the solution until the ringworm is cleared completely.

Mustard Seed – can aid in the treatment of ringworm. Simply take powdered mustard seed and mix it with water. Stir the mixture until it forms a thick paste. Once the paste has formed apply it to the affected area of skin. You will want to leave the paste on the ringworm for at least 30-35 minutes. You can then wash the affected area with cool water.

Turmeric – this is a very powerful treatment for ringworm and can be all performed in the comforts of your own home. Taking the juice from fresh raw turmeric can not only help with the fight against the fungal infection but can also clear the ringworm in little to no time. You can use this home remedy as an oral treatment or by applying a mixture to the affected area. To make the oral solution, simply take one teaspoon on turmeric juice and mix it with a teaspoon of honey. Take this mixture very morning until the fungal infection is cleared. To use this home remedy as a mixture to apply to the affected skin, simply apply the turmeric juice directly to the ringworm. You will see results very quickly and can also be used in the prevention of ringworm in early stages.

Aloe Vera – this is very well-known for the treatment of many different skin conditions, even ringworm. You can use Aloe Vera gel or by taking Aloe Vera directly from the plant. Aloe Vera not only heals the affected area of skin but also alleviates any of the itching sensations due to the fungal infection. Apply the Aloe Vera very generously throughout the day and repeat the process until the fungal infection is completely cleared up.

Spinach and Carrot Juice – both have properties to help kill many types of fungal infections, ringworm in particular. Simply mix equal parts of spinach juice and carrot juice and apply the mixture to the affected area or areas. Do this several times during the day until the ringworm is completely cleared.

Lemon and Lime – also work hand in hand in the treatment of ringworm. Simply squeeze half of a lime and half of a lemon into a dish. Soak a clean cloth or towel with the mixture and apply it to the affected area. You should follow this procedure at least 2 times a day. This can potentially treat the fungal infection in less than a week.

Apple Cider Vinegar – This is also a very well-known and commonly used home remedy for ringworm. Simply soak a cotton ball or band-aid in the apple cider vinegar and then apply it to the affected area. Make sure to keep this on the affected area and reapply at least 2-3 times a day. This is a fast acting home remedy that can also have your ringworm cleared up and gone in just a couple of nights.

Potato Slices – You may also want to try another popular home remedy that involves potato slices. Simply apply a slice of a potato on the affected area every night before bed. You may want to tape the potato slice to the area of affected skin so that it can constantly be on the ringworm the whole time you are sleeping. Doing this home remedy you can expect to see results in as little as 2-3 days.

Goldenseal Powder – is also a home remedy that can clear up many fungal infections including ringworm. Simply take a small amount of goldenseal powder and apply it to water. Mix until a thick paste has formed. Apply the paste directly to the affected area and allow the paste to dry. Perform this home remedy several times during the day until the fungal infection is completely cleared up.

Iodine – This is another home remedy that people have found to clear up ringworm. Simply apply iodine to the affected areas of skin and allow it to dry. You will need to apply the iodine at least 3 times a day. Within days you will see your fungal infection completely diminished.

Tea Tree Oil – can also be applied to the affected area by soaking a cotton ball or q-tip in the tea tree oil and then applying it to the affected areas of skin. You will however need to dilute with a small amount of water.

Papaya – Cut slices of papaya and place it on the affected area of skin. Leave the slices on the affected area for at least 10-20 minutes. Direct pulp contact is the key.

Sore Throat

A sore throat can be a very painful and irritating condition for many people. There are many symptoms associated with a sore throat such as loss of voice, redness, dryness, coughing, clogged nasal passages, and swallowing difficulty. Although there are many home remedies you can try to ease your symptoms from a sore throat you will need to keep in mind that a sore throat can also lead to more prolonged illnesses if not treated properly. When using these home remedies if your sore throat does not subside within 3-4 days of using the remedies, or if you start having a fever, you need to contact your primary physician and schedule an appointment to come in. Strep throat is very common amongst people and children and if left untreated can turn into Scarlett fever, a very dangerous and possible life threatening illness. Below are a few home remedies you can try before rushing to the doctor with sore throat symptoms.

Useful Treatment Tips

> ➤ Take a cup of beet juice and add two tablespoons of honey. Mix the two ingredients together and heat it up for about one minute. Gently drink the solution for about 15 minutes.

> ➤ You can also make some tea using powdered ginger and water. Simply add half of a teaspoon of ground cayenne pepper with your brewing tea also and you have now created an herbal tea that will have your throat feeling a world of difference. Keep in mind to

keep stirring the mixture as the pepper will settle. For best results drink this home remedy before bedtime. This mixture is also very handy when it comes to curing an irritating cough.

➢ You can also try fresh pure squeezed lemon juice. Lemons contain citric acid which can help relieve swollen parts, hence your irritated and sore throat.

➢ Taking a shot of whisky or tequila with a tablespoon of honey can also relieve most sore throats. Let the mixture sit in the back of your throat for at least 15-20 seconds and then swallow the mixture to sure your sore and aching throat.

➢ You can also try heating a cup of milk and adding a teaspoon of butter and honey. You can also sprinkle sugar for a better tasting mixture.

➢ Lemon herbal tea with chamomile can also be a cure for your sore throat. You can also mix in honey to add to your sore throat infusion. Simply boil the mixture and then gently sip the concoction.

➢ Who could forget old fashioned salt and water? Simply ad one to two tablespoons of salt to warm water and gargle the mixture for several minutes.

➢ Ginger is also a very effective home remedy for sore throats. You can either consume ginger through tea form or it can be made into a hot beverage or with plain water and sugar. The juice of ginger can also be taken with honey to treat a sore throat.

- By adding cumin seeds to boiling water and then adding garlic can also be a great mixture to mix up with you have the sore throat blues. After boiling the mixture you will then want to simmer the concoction and allow it to cool. Consume the mixture in a timely matter will determine on the effectiveness of the concoction.

- An infusion of cinnamon and cardamom can also be gargled and can treat your aching sore throat. This is also used to help with sore throats associated with the flu.

- Licorice is also a great ingredient to help cure sore throats. Simply suck on pieces of raw licorice and allow the juices to pass through your throat to help soothing the redness and irritation of your throat.

- By filling a cup with honey and adding onion pieces. After making the mixture you can swallow one teaspoon of the mixture each and every two hours for instant relief for a sore throat.

- Another effective way to cure a sore throat is mango bark chewing.

- Belleric myrobalan is a fruit, however it is not the fruit that you need for your sore throat concoction but the pulp of the fruit. What you want to do is take the pulp of its fruit and mix it with salt, pepper, and honey.

- Pouring one cup of boiling water over two teaspoons of dried raspberry leaves and steep them for ten minutes. After straining the mixture allow it to cool and then gargle the mixture.

➤ You can also try mixing a cup of warm water with a teaspoon of turmeric powder and a half of a teaspoon of salt. Mix this all together and gargle the mixture 2-3 times a day.

➤ Mixing a teaspoon of sage in a cup of boiling water can also do the trick for a sore throat. After straining the mixture and allowing it to cool you can then add one teaspoon of honey and a teaspoon of apple cider vinegar. Gargle the mixture 3-4 times a day.

➤ Gargling Listerine is also a very effective method for curing a sore throat.

Sunburn

People can always find fun in the sun... except when they get too much sun. Sunburns can be one of the most miserable conditions to have because it can affect huge amounts of your body... especially if you have been out in the sun in a bathing suit. Not only is a sunburn painful but it also makes it uncomfortable to sleep, wear clothing, or even touching or rubbing the skin. However, there are some home remedies that can help you with treating and catering to your symptoms from sunburns. Below are the top home remedies that have been tested and proven to help with sunburn conditions and pain.

Milk – has been used for many years to treat sunburns. The lactic acid and fat that is found in milk are properties that are known to have soothing qualities for sunburned skin. In this home remedy you will want to soak a soft cloth or towel in cool milk. After the cloth or towel has been soaked you want to carefully apply it onto the areas that are sunburned. Follow this procedure for 15-20 minutes and then rinse off with cool water. Make sure that the milk that you are using is whole milk, due to the amount of fat it contains compared to skim or 2% milk. The amount of fat found in the milk does make a difference in the effect of this home remedy.

Aloe Vera – has to be the most effective and most common home remedy used for sunburns. Aloe Vera not only gives your skin soothing pain relief but also helps in the treatment of your sunburn. You can take the gel extract from an Aloe Vera plant directly or you can also find Aloe Vera gel at your local pharmacy. Make sure that when purchasing over the counter Aloe Vera gel or cream that it contains a high concentration of Aloe Vera than it does water or other solutions. However, the most effective form is using the gel extract straight from an Aloe Vera plant. Simply apply the gel to the affected area and use the gel as needed for pain relief until the sunburn subsides.

Water – can also help you with pain relief as well as the treatment of sunburns. When using water in a home remedy always remember to use cold water. Your skin is already burnt and does not need any more heat applied to it than it already has. There are a couple of different things that you do to you can do during bath time that will help with your sunburn symptoms. You can simply take a cold bath keeping the affected areas submerged under water for 15-20 minutes. If the areas underneath your eyes and cheeks are affected you can take slices of cucumbers, tomatoes, or potatoes, or tea bags can be applied to help with pain and healing. You can also add a half of a teaspoon of vinegar to a bucket of cold water. Soak either a soft cloth or towel in the mixture and apply it directly to the affected areas. You can also use equal parts of water and milk and get the same effects for sunburn relief. Another great home remedy using cold bath water is by adding 5-6 tablespoons of oatmeal to a cold bath. Keep your body submerged in the cool water and oatmeal for around 15-20 minutes. Not only will this method reduce the irritation of the skin but also helps treat and heal the sunburn also. You may also want to try using a few drops of peppermint oil and adding it to your coo bath water for instant pain relief.

Cucumber Juice – is very powerful in the fight against inflammation and redness to the skin. It also moisturizes the damaged skin and replenishes the new skin post sunburn. In this home remedy you take a tablespoon of cucumber juice and mix it with a tablespoon of milk. Soak a towel or soft cloth with the solution and then apply it to the affected areas. You can find cucumber juice at your local grocery or nutritional store.

Lettuce and Cabbage – These are both natural and beneficial home remedies that can help treat your sunburn. Simply take refrigerated lettuce or cabbage leaves and apply them to the skin that is affected. Almost instantly you should feel relief and helps in the healing process.

Sugarless Tea – is also a great home remedy that helps soothe and relieve the pain and discomfort to the affected skin. The reason for this is because tea has an active ingredient of tannin. Simply brew some tea and allow it to cool. After the tea has cooled completely you will then want to take either a soft towel or cloth and soak it with the tea. Dab the areas of skin that are affected from the sunburn. Be sure to keep the used teabags because you can use these for the more sensitive areas such as the eyes.

Useful Treatment Tips

> You may also want to try rubbing mustard oil on the burnt areas of the skin. After you have rubbed all

affected areas, allow the mustard oil to dry. This can take away a lot of the heat due to the sunburn.

➤ You can also apply sandalwood paste to the affected areas of skin. This has been used for many years to relieve the pain and discomfort due to sunburns.

➤ Mixing one part tomato juice and six parts buttermilk to affected areas of skin can not only help with the pain and discomfort but also helps heal the burns themselves. Allow the mixture to dry. Then wash the mixture of after 25-30 minutes.

➤ Another well-known home remedy for sunburn relief is doing Epsom salt compressions to the affected areas of skin and watch your sunburn symptoms diminish

Thyroid Problems

Hyperthyroidism and Hypothyroidism

There are two types of thyroid conditions, hyperthyroidism which is when your thyroid glands become overly active and produces more hormones than are required, and hypothyroidism which is when your thyroid glands are working below average and doesn't produce enough hormones that average thyroid glands produce. There are different home remedies that you can use for each and both are conditions that will need to be treated for proper thyroid function. Be sure that you are having your levels thyroid levels checked periodically. Keep a record of your TSH (thyroid stimulating hormone) levels and see what home remedies work best for you and your body.

Hyperthyroidism

Iodine – This can be a very effective home remedy to use when treating hyperthyroidism because iodine is what your thyroid glands need to function properly. You can get iodine supplements at your local drug store and will need to contain tablets that are 225mcg. You will also want to consume foods that are high in iodine to take with your iodine supplements. Foods that are high in iodine are foods such as seafood, bananas, eggs, meat, yogurt, oatmeal, and potatoes. Also using iodized salt instead of using sea salt can also benefit lowering your thyroid levels. Using iodine in your diet will naturally and effectively decrease your thyroid levels dramatically. Try consuming iodine food items as well as a iodine supplement daily and watch your levels now regularly in the normal average range.

Tyrosine - Tyrosine is responsible for producing thyroid hormones that come from iodine and are also a very important amino acid that your body needs. You can find tyrosine from your local drug store and is a dietary supplement. For best results make sure to incorporate this into your meal plans daily.

Bladderwrack – this is traditionally used to help the treatment of weight loss which is caused by thyroid problems. Bladderwrack is a type of seaweed that has high levels of iodine. You can find bladderwrack in your local drug store and can be bought in food supplement form or it can also be cooked into your brewing tea. Both ways are effective and also help increase your metabolism.

Coconut Oil -   Consuming a few tablespoons daily, preferably one tablespoon after each meal can help lower your overly active thyroid glands. This is an essential oil that can help maintain a good metabolism and can also cure from an excessive weight loss. You can also use coconut oil in your meals and also find your thyroid levels dropping at your next visit to the doctor.

Lemon Balm – is also a good herb that helps reduce your overly active thyroid levels naturally. You consume lemon balm by brewing it with your tea. Substituting lemon balm tea with your coffee or any other caffeinated drink will help lower your thyroid levels almost instantly and can lower levels up to 10 percent.

Antioxidants – Antioxidants can also help manage the excessive hormone production that your thyroid glands are producing. Antioxidants such as Vitamin C and green tea can be used to flush your body as well as flush your blood from any unwanted and unneeded chemicals that can be found inside your body. You can find Vitamin C capsules at your local drug store and can be found in foods such as juices and citrus fruits. Consuming Vitamin C as well as green teas at least two times daily will keep your levels free from any progression of your hyperthyroidism.

Motherwort Herb – This is a type of herb that has been used for centuries and was originally used for the cure of depression and heart palpitations. However, more recent studies have shown that it also helps cure hyperthyroidism. Motherwort herb decreases the activity in the thyroid gland that is causing the increased production of hormones. Brewing a tea with this herb or being used as a food supplement are both very effective methods for consuming the herb. Consume motherwort herb at least one time a day and you will see your thyroid levels decrease by an astounding 15 percent.

Dandelion Root – Using the roots of dandelions as an ingredient for your tea can also help lower your thyroid levels and the activity of your thyroid glands. Simply boil the roots with water and then add the mixture to your tea. You can consume this mixture one to two times a day for an effective method to naturally regulate your overly stimulated thyroid glands.

Hypothyroidism

Spirulina – This herb is a very good source to use to increase the productivity of hormones by your thyroid glands. This herb also helps regulate thyroid glands and give them a boost of good health. You can find spirulina at your local drug store or nutritional supplement stores. Incorporating this herb brewed with your tea can be a very effective way to increase your thyroid levels and function.

Black Cohosh – This is another well-known herb that has been tested and proven to increase the function of your thyroid glands as well balances out levels of estrogen in women. Brewing this herb with your tea is a great way to consume this herb and very effective. You can also find food supplements that contain this particular herb and has also been proven to be an effective treatment for hypothyroidism.

Primrose Oil – Primrose oil contains the proper amount of fatty acids that is essential for the functioning of your thyroid as well as for good health all around. Again this oil can be found in pill form as well as through a food supplement. Incorporating this handy ingredient daily can help increase your thyroid levels quickly and effectively.

Agnus Castus – Many people aren't aware that abnormal estrogen levels can alter the functioning of the thyroid glands. By using angus castus you can not only bring these levels back to the normal range but also can help improve the function of the pituitary gland. Check with your local drug store or nutritional store for more details on the availability of this helpful method.

Mullein – also helps to cover and protect cells as well as reduce inflammation of your thyroid glands. This is a very handy method if you have a goiter also.

Vitamin B Complex – the regular intake of a vitamin B complex capsule can also greatly help your thyroid condition and proper function. Another great plus to takng a vitamin B complex is that it can also help prevent from other minor diseases. Along with taking a vitamin B complex you will also want to incorporate the consumption of green leafy vegetables. Vitamin B complex also improves cell oxygenation and can help increase your energy. Not only does it help increase the productivity of your thyroid but it also helps with immunity and rejuvenated your body also.

Useful Treatment Tips

> Consuming foods like cabbage, broccoli, radishes, cauliflower, and turnips can dramatically help the function of your thyroid glands whether you have hyperthyroidism or hypothyroidism. Although keep in mind that if you have hypothyroidism you will not want to take in too much of these items because consuming large amounts of these types of foods can also increase thyroid function.

➤ You will want to reduce your intake of sugar, dairy, caffeine, and alcohol. You will also want to reduce the amount of carbs and fats that you eat to decrease the amount of calories that you are taking in per day.

➤ With thyroid conditions a person most commonly also has to deal with weight issues. Pepper is a great source for increasing and normalizing your metabolism which in turn helps normalize your weight also.

➤ Regular intake of foods that are rich in magnesium, iron, zinc, calcium, neodymium, copper, manganese, and terbium can also help a healthy functioning thyroid.

➤ Cayenne, ginger, and kelp can also help with inadequate weight due to the dysfunction of your thyroid glands.

Toothache

A toothache can be a very painful experience for anyone to have to suffer with. On top of all that many people fear going to the dentist. Keep in mind that most of the time the reason for a person getting a toothache is either due to an infection or a problem with the tooth or jaw. For that reason if your toothache is persistent for more than 3 or 4 days you will need to consult with your dentist. Another big sign to head on over to the dentist is if a fever is incorporated with the toothache. This is another sign of infection and could turn into a life threatening condition also. However, there are some natural home remedies that you can try to ease the pain and discomfort experienced by a toothache. Below are the top natural home remedies that have been used for many years and have been tested and proven to help with the symptoms associated with a toothache.

Useful Treatment Tips

> ➤ Garlic is a very common and very effective home remedy to use to help with your toothache pain. Using a clove of garlic mixed with rock salt and then placed on the affected tooth can bring your tooth instant relief. Sometimes this very home remedy can even cure your toothache. You can also try chewing a garlic clove, preferably in the morning and then periodically through the day when the toothache pain starts to persist.

➤ Another useful home remedy to help with your aches and pains of a tooth is by taking a small piece of onion and placing it on the sore tooth or gum. Onions have antibacterial properties and will not only help ease the pain of your aching tooth but also help kill germs and bacteria present in the affected tooth and the mouth.

➤ You can also take drops of vanilla extract and apply them to the affected tooth for instant relief in pain and a very effective home remedy to cure your toothache.

➤ An old home remedy that has been used for ages is by mixing some pepper powder with table salt and then rubbing the mixture on the affected tooth. This home remedy can also be useful if used daily. By using this method daily it helps with the prevention of any reoccurring toothaches as well as prevents against any cavities forming in the tooth.

➤ Another great home remedy for curing your toothache blues is by melting 1 teaspoon of baking soda in a glass of water. After mixing the two ingredients you can then use the mixture as a mouth wash. This cleans away infection in both the tooth and the mouth. Keep in mind infection is the leading source to pain.

➤ You may also want to try taking turmeric sticks and burning them making them a fine powder. Place the powder on the aching tooth and can see almost instant relief to your tooth pain.

➢ Limes are also a very powerful preventative as can also help with pains associated with toothaches. Limes can prevent against cavities, bleeding of gums, tooth decay, and also any loosening of the teeth.

➢ You may also want to try taking Asafoetida grounded; and mixing it into lemon juice. Simply take the mixture and heat. After the mixture has warmed, you can then take a cotton swab and soak it with the mixture. Rub the cotton swab on the affected tooth and you will find that you now have instant relief from your aching tooth.

➢ Another great home remedy you can try is mixing the bark of bay berry and some vinegar. Take a cotton swab and soak it in the mixture and then rub the cotton swab on the affected tooth. This will not only help alleviate tooth pain, but also helps strengthen your gums.

➢ One of the most popular home remedies for a toothache is clove. Clove consists of clove oil, which helps in the relief of pain almost instantly, and also contains properties of antiseptics. If you don't have any clove oil you can also grind up a clove and then apply the powder on the affected tooth. This natural home remedy has been used for hundreds of years and has been proven to help reduce the pain you suffer associated with a toothache.

➢ Using the oil of oregano can also provide you with instant toothache pain.

➢ Drinking the juice of a star fruit can also help get relief to your aching tooth. Simply consume the juice at least two times a day and you will be surprised at the relief you get, from such a tasty juice.

➢ You can also create a very powerful mouthwash by taking the juice of wheat grass that not only helps to prevent tooth decay but also has been proven to cure most common toothaches. The wheat draws out toxins that are present in your gums and helps prevent against any growth of bacteria in the mouth and teeth.

Urinary Tract Infection

A urinary tract infection, or UTI, is a very painful, uncomfortable, and irritating infection to have. UTI's most commonly affect more women than men. A UTI is a bacterial infection that is most commonly started with E-coli entering the bladder. Although some infections can be present in a bladder and the body naturally flushes it out, there are occurrences where there is a backup of infection, therefore causing a person to have a UTI. There are many ways to treat a UTI and many find that home remedies work better and clear up UTI's faster and more effectively than prescriptions. Another staggering note is that over 25% of people that use prescriptions to clear up their UTI symptoms have a reoccurring UTI within a few months, proving that home remedies are the way to go when it comes to treating your UTI symptoms. Note that if your symptoms persist for more than 5-7 days after home treatment has been used that you will need to contact your regular physician for further conditions. Here are a few home remedies that you can try to help cure common symptoms associated with UTI's.

Useful Treatment Tips

> One of the most popular forms of curing a UTI is by drinking unsweetened cranberry juice. Drinking unsweetened cranberry juice regularly can also help fight against E-coli bacteria from forming in your bladder. For best results you will want to consume at least 4-6 glasses per day when you are suffering from a UTI. Drinking 1-2 glasses each day when

you don't have a UTI will successfully prevent you from recurrent UTI's in the future.

➤ You may also want to try using alfalfa in your treatment plan for your UTI symptoms. You can buy alfalfa in the form of juice concentrate and can rid toxins from your body, bladder, and urinary tract, as well as increases the flow of urine. The alfalfa juice helps improve kidney function, which is a must when trying to fight off infections in your urinary tract and bladder. You can also try incorporating both alfalfa juice and cranberry extract tablets and get a double dose of fighting for your UTI.

➤ Another great home remedy for helping you with your UTI symptoms is Zinc and Vitamin C. You can find these supplements at your local pharmacy and at nutritional stores also. Normally a person should take 3000 mg of Vitamin C and 3 Zinc lozenges per day to fight off their UTI. Zinc and Vitamin C booth help boost your immune system as well as helps fight off bacterial infections quickly.

➤ You can also try drinking a mixture of a half of a teaspoon of baking soda in a glass of water when your symptoms of a UTI first start to occur. This can prevent a UTI from even forming.

➤ You need to also increase your water intake dramatically during a UTI. This means drinking a minimum of 8-10 glasses per day. Water is the most effective and natural way to flush out your entire body of bacteria. The quicker you are able to flush out bacteria in your bladder and urinary tract the faster your symptoms will subside.

➤ Another great way to reduce the pain and discomfort from a UTI is by placing a heating pad or even a hot water bottle covered by a towel, and placing it on your abdomen. The heat will provide you with pain relief due to associated UTI symptoms.

➤ There are also certain fruits and vegetables that have been proven to flush out your body and helps rid your body with bad bacteria from forming. During the course of your UTI you will want to make sure that some of the foods listed are used in your meal plan. The fruits and vegetables included are green beans, apples, carrots, squash, grapes, pears, broccoli, onions, potatoes, spinach, avocados, and zucchini.

➤ Keep in mind that during the course of your UTI that you avoid wearing tight undergarments or jeans. Make sure to wear only cotton underwear and don't use perfumed products in your vaginal area as this will cause more irritation.

➤ Make sure that even though it may be hard and painful to urinate, that you don't resist your urge to urinate. Remember that you are trying to get rid of the bacteria that formed in your bladder and the only true way to get rid of the bacteria is through urination. The more frequent flow of urination you have during the course of a UTI the faster the bacteria can be cleansed from the bladder and urinary tract, the faster you will get to the road of recovery from your UTI.

Yeast Infections

Statistics show that women, in particular, will have at least one yeast infection in their life. Although yeast infections can occur in men, women are notably the most common victims to a yeast infection. A yeast infection is a fungus that forms when the good bacteria is taken over by bad bacteria. The good bacteria present in your body helps balance the yeast, so when the good bacteria are taken over bad bacteria; yeast starts to build and forms a yeast infection. This is a very painful and uncomfortable condition and can actually be caused by prescription antibiotics also. Some women will find themselves with a yeast infection after the duration of their antibiotics. This is why most women find themselves turning to home remedies to cure their yeast infections first before running to the doctor. Here are a few of the tops home remedies you can use to help your yeast infection symptoms quickly and effectively.

Garlic – is one of the most powerful and most effective sources to killing yeast present in the body. This home remedy has been used for many years and has since been tested and proven to really work and actually clears up a yeast infection. You will need garlic cloves or garlic tablets, which can be picked up at your local pharmacy or nutritional store. Now, this may sound crazy, but you insert one garlic tablet or one garlic clove into the vagina every few hours or on an as needed basis to soothe the pain. Another remedy that you can use with garlic is taking a clove of garlic and crushing it, then place the crushed garlic in a boiling cup of water. Let the mixture boil around 10-15 minutes and then strain the garlic. Consume the garlic water while the mixture is lukewarm. Garlic is used to cure a lot of conditions and illnesses and will help you greatly in the treatment of a yeast infection. Garlic acts as a natural antibiotic and fights against bad bacteria and yeast also.

Apple Cider Vinegar – Another great home remedy that helps with the treatment of a yeast infection is apple cider vinegar. Apple cider vinegar kills yeast and has been tested and proven to also help with pain relief from the symptoms of a yeast infection. Simply take about a cup of apple cider vinegar and place it in a lukewarm bath. Relax and lay in the nice warm bath for about 20 minutes. This can not only help clear up a yeast infection but relaxes you and soothes your pain from the yeast infection.

Yogurt - has properties of good bacteria and good bacteria is what fights off yeast... so why not load your body up with good bacteria to help treat a yeast infection. However, it does matter on what type of yogurt you consume. It is the plain yogurt that is unsweetened that contain the most properties of good bacteria. Sugar only feeds yeast, so it is very important that the yogurt that you consume has no sugar added. Consuming a cup of yogurt at least 2-3 times a day will help immensely with the pain and treatment of a yeast infection. You can also try your hand at making your own homemade yogurt. This holds a great benefit because when you make your own yogurt you can choose what type of milk to use and using soy or almond milk greatly helps in   destroying   unwanted   yeast   in   your   body.

Tea Tree Oil – can also be used in a home remedy for yeast infections. First you will want to mix the tea tree oil with rubbing alcohol. You then want to take a dropper and fill it with the solution and then insert and apply the solution to the affected area internally. You can also use a tampon if you prefer by soaking the tampon in the mixture and then inserting the tampon into the affected area. If you are using the tampon method make sure to only leave the tampon inserted for at least 2 hours. You can apply the mixture 1-2 times a day and until the course of the yeast infection has subsided. This also helps with the soothing the pain due to the symptoms of the yeast infection.

Useful Treatment Tips

> ➤ You can also try mixing olive leaf extract with some grape fruit seed extract in a glass of water and consume the mixture 2-3 times a day. Both of the extracts help fight against infection and yeast as well. Another great home remedy that you can try that involves extracts is taking a cranberry extract or a cranberry blueberry extract and mix it with a glass of water. You can also consume this mixture 2-3 times a day. These two extracts also work as good antioxidants along with the fight against yeast.

> ➤ You may also want to try drinking at least 2 glasses of buttermilk per day. This home remedy can not only help in the treatment of a yeast infection but also can act as a preventive one if you have yeast infections that are reoccurring. Incorporate plain yogurt and a glass of buttermilk for the treatment of

your yeast infection and watch your symptoms drift away.

➤ Another great home remedy that is very effective in the treatment of a yeast infection is by applying baby oil that has Aloe Vera and Vitamin E in it to the affected area. This will not only sooth the irritation due to the yeast infection and will also reduce the itching symptom caused by the yeast infection.

➤ During the course of the yeast infection make sure to wear loose fighting jeans or bottoms and only cotton underwear. This will reduce a lot of unneeded irritation.

Conclusion

So there you have it… all the top home remedies for your most common illnesses and conditions. The best part is, you are receiving treatment for your symptoms through the more natural and beneficial way possible… through home remedies.

No more filling your body with unwanted medication that can only harm you and your organs in the end. No more never ending side effects. Many of the home remedies mentioned in this book can also act as double aids to many different illnesses and conditions.

Like I have said before, make sure that if your symptoms do not clear up within 5-7 days of your symptoms starting that you contact your physician for further treatment. You will also want to make sure that you are not allergic to any of the ingredients or substances used in the home remedies. You may also want to check with your physician if you suffer from multiple conditions to make sure that each home remedy is right for you.

You can also check online for other home remedies for your illness or condition. There are many home remedies for many different illnesses and conditions and new home remedies are discovered every day.

I have uncovered many home remedies for the top illnesses and conditions such as high blood pressure, gout, the common cold, sore throat, allergies, psoriasis, ringworm, and even a hangover, along with the many home remedies to clear the symptoms associated with that particular illness or condition.

Note that all of the ingredients can be found at any pharmacy or nutritional store locally, so there is no need to panic. You can also ask your local pharmacist for recommendations on over the counter remedies for your particular illness or condition.

I hope that this book has been beneficial and helps you in your home remedy search for your illness or condition. Remember that these are only the top remedies; there are many other remedies so do some research for many others. Herbal home remedies also are very beneficial in balancing a normal and balanced body as well as treats many different conditions.

Share your new-found remedies to your family and friends... they will be glad you did and will find them using home remedies rather than prescription medications also. So start using home remedies and you will find a better more effective and beneficial way treat the most common illnesses and conditions today!

Additional Resources

LearningHerbs.com - Lots of great information on herbs and making your own home remedies.
http://www.learningherbs.com/

Native Remedies - Provides a wide range of proven, safe and effective herbal remedies for People and Pets.
http://thekitchenherbalist.com/NativeRemedies.htm

New Body Herbs Online - Provide purely organic herbs and herbal formulas.
http://thekitchenherbalist.com/NewBodyHerbs.htm

Herbal Remedies - Over 5,000 of the finest natural health supplements and herbal products available!
http://thekitchenherbalist.com/HerbalRemedies.htm

Penn Herb Company - Most places only sell herbs in supplement form. This is a good place to buy dried herbs in bulk if you want to experiment with your own herbal recipes and teas.
http://www.pennherb.com/

Printed in Great Britain
by Amazon.co.uk, Ltd.,
Marston Gate.